MY QUOTABLE PATIENTS

THE FUNNIEST THINGS MY PATIENTS SAY

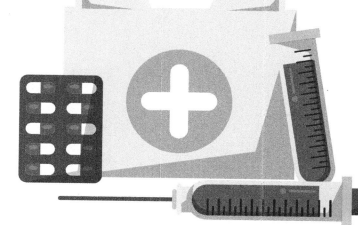

THIS BELONGS TO:

_____

FUNNY MEMORIES

Who: _____	When: _____
To: _____	With: _____

Story/Situation

_____

_____

_____

_____

_____

What Was Said

_____

_____

_____

_____

_____

_____

What I Said/My Initial Reaction

_____

_____

_____

_____

_____

_____

What I Wish I Said

_____

_____

_____

_____

_____

_____

_____

_____

FUNNY MEMORIES

Who: _____	When: _____
To: _____	With: _____

Story/Situation

_____

_____

_____

_____

_____

What Was Said

_____

_____

_____

_____

_____

_____

What I Said/My Initial Reaction

_____

_____

_____

_____

_____

_____

What I Wish I Said

_____

_____

_____

_____

_____

_____

_____

_____

FUNNY MEMORIES

Who: _____   When: _____

To: _____   With: _____

Story/Situation

_____

_____

_____

_____

_____

What Was Said

_____

_____

_____

_____

_____

_____

_____

What I Said/My Initial Reaction

_____

_____

_____

_____

_____

_____

What I Wish I Said

_____

_____

_____

_____

_____

_____

_____

_____

FUNNY MEMORIES

Who:_____	When: _____
To:_____	With: _____

Story/Situation

_____

_____

_____

_____

_____

What Was Said

_____

_____

_____

_____

_____

_____

What I Said/My Initial Reaction

_____

_____

_____

_____

_____

_____

What I Wish I Said

_____

_____

_____

_____

_____

_____

_____

_____

FUNNY MEMORIES

| Who: _____ | When: _____ |
| To: _____ | With: _____ |

Story/Situation

_____

_____

_____

_____

_____

What Was Said

_____

_____

_____

_____

_____

_____

_____

What I Said/My Initial Reaction

_____

_____

_____

_____

_____

_____

What I Wish I Said

_____

_____

_____

_____

_____

_____

_____

_____

FUNNY MEMORIES

Who: _____	When: _____
To: _____	With: _____

Story/Situation

_____

_____

_____

_____

_____

What Was Said

_____

_____

_____

_____

_____

_____

_____

What I Said/My Initial Reaction

_____

_____

_____

_____

_____

_____

What I Wish I Said

_____

_____

_____

_____

_____

_____

_____

_____

FUNNY MEMORIES

Who:_____   When:_____

To:_____   With:_____

Story/Situation

_____

_____

_____

_____

_____

What Was Said

_____

_____

_____

_____

_____

_____

What I Said/My Initial Reaction

_____

_____

_____

_____

_____

_____

What I Wish I Said

_____

_____

_____

_____

_____

_____

_____

_____

_____

FUNNY MEMORIES

Who: _____

When: _____

To: _____

With: _____

Story/Situation

_____

_____

_____

_____

_____

What Was Said

_____

_____

_____

_____

_____

_____

What I Said/My Initial Reaction

_____

_____

_____

_____

_____

_____

What I Wish I Said

_____

_____

_____

_____

_____

_____

_____

_____

FUNNY MEMORIES

| Who: _____ | When: _____ |
| To: _____ | With: _____ |

Story/Situation

_____

_____

_____

_____

_____

What Was Said

_____

_____

_____

_____

_____

_____

What I Said/My Initial Reaction

_____

_____

_____

_____

_____

_____

What I Wish I Said

_____

_____

_____

_____

_____

_____

_____

_____

_____

FUNNY MEMORIES

| Who: _____ | When: _____ |
| To: _____ | With: _____ |

Story/Situation

_____

_____

_____

_____

_____

What Was Said

_____

_____

_____

_____

_____

_____

What I Said/My Initial Reaction

_____

_____

_____

_____

_____

_____

What I Wish I Said

_____

_____

_____

_____

_____

_____

_____

_____

_____

FUNNY MEMORIES

Who:_____	When:_____
To:_____	With:_____

Story/Situation

_____

_____

_____

_____

_____

What Was Said

_____

_____

_____

_____

_____

_____

What I Said/My Initial Reaction

_____

_____

_____

_____

_____

_____

What I Wish I Said

_____

_____

_____

_____

_____

_____

_____

_____

FUNNY MEMORIES

| Who: _____ | When: _____ |
| To: _____ | With: _____ |

Story/Situation

_____

_____

_____

_____

_____

What Was Said

_____

_____

_____

_____

_____

_____

_____

What I Said/My Initial Reaction

_____

_____

_____

_____

_____

_____

What I Wish I Said

_____

_____

_____

_____

_____

_____

_____

FUNNY MEMORIES

Who:_____	When:_____
To:_____	With:_____

Story/Situation

_____

_____

_____

_____

_____

What Was Said

_____

_____

_____

_____

_____

_____

What I Said/My Initial Reaction

_____

_____

_____

_____

_____

_____

What I Wish I Said

_____

_____

_____

_____

_____

_____

_____

_____

_____

FUNNY MEMORIES

Who: _____	When: _____
To: _____	With: _____

Story/Situation

_____

_____

_____

_____

_____

What Was Said

_____

_____

_____

_____

_____

_____

What I Said/My Initial Reaction

_____

_____

_____

_____

_____

_____

What I Wish I Said

_____

_____

_____

_____

_____

_____

_____

_____

FUNNY MEMORIES

Who: _____   **When:** _____

To: _____   **With:** _____

Story/Situation

_____

_____

_____

_____

_____

What Was Said

_____

_____

_____

_____

_____

_____

What I Said/My Initial Reaction

_____

_____

_____

_____

_____

_____

What I Wish I Said

_____

_____

_____

_____

_____

_____

_____

_____

_____

FUNNY MEMORIES

Who: _____

When: _____

To: _____

With: _____

Story/Situation

_____

_____

_____

_____

_____

What Was Said

_____

_____

_____

_____

_____

_____

What I Said/My Initial Reaction

_____

_____

_____

_____

_____

What I Wish I Said

_____

_____

_____

_____

_____

_____

_____

_____

FUNNY MEMORIES

Who: _____   When: _____

To: _____   With: _____

Story/Situation

_____

_____

_____

_____

_____

What Was Said

_____

_____

_____

_____

_____

_____

_____

What I Said/My Initial Reaction

_____

_____

_____

_____

_____

_____

What I Wish I Said

_____

_____

_____

_____

_____

_____

_____

_____

FUNNY MEMORIES

Who: _____

When: _____

To: _____

With: _____

Story/Situation

_____

_____

_____

_____

_____

What Was Said

_____

_____

_____

_____

_____

_____

_____

What I Said/My Initial Reaction

_____

_____

_____

_____

_____

What I Wish I Said

_____

_____

_____

_____

_____

_____

_____

FUNNY MEMORIES

Who: _____   When: _____

To: _____   With: _____

Story/Situation

_____

_____

_____

_____

_____

What Was Said

_____

_____

_____

_____

_____

_____

_____

What I Said/My Initial Reaction

_____

_____

_____

_____

_____

_____

What I Wish I Said

_____

_____

_____

_____

_____

_____

_____

_____

_____

FUNNY MEMORIES

Who: _____   **When:** _____

To: _____   **With:** _____

Story/Situation

_____

_____

_____

_____

_____

What Was Said

_____

_____

_____

_____

_____

_____

_____

What I Said/My Initial Reaction

_____

_____

_____

_____

_____

_____

What I Wish I Said

_____

_____

_____

_____

_____

_____

_____

_____

FUNNY MEMORIES

Who: _____ **When:** _____

To: _____ **With:** _____

Story/Situation

_____

_____

_____

_____

_____

What Was Said

_____

_____

_____

_____

_____

_____

_____

What I Said/My Initial Reaction

_____

_____

_____

_____

_____

_____

What I Wish I Said

_____

_____

_____

_____

_____

_____

_____

_____

_____

_____

FUNNY MEMORIES

Who: _____	When: _____
To: _____	With: _____

Story/Situation

_____

_____

_____

_____

_____

What Was Said

_____

_____

_____

_____

_____

_____

What I Said/My Initial Reaction

_____

_____

_____

_____

_____

_____

What I Wish I Said

_____

_____

_____

_____

_____

_____

_____

_____

FUNNY MEMORIES

| Who: _____ | When: _____ |
| To: _____ | With: _____ |

Story/Situation

_____

_____

_____

_____

_____

What Was Said

_____

_____

_____

_____

_____

_____

_____

What I Said/My Initial Reaction

_____

_____

_____

_____

_____

_____

What I Wish I Said

_____

_____

_____

_____

_____

_____

_____

_____

FUNNY MEMORIES

Who: _____ **When:** _____

To: _____ **With:** _____

Story/Situation

_____

_____

_____

_____

_____

What Was Said

_____

_____

_____

_____

_____

_____

_____

What I Said/My Initial Reaction

_____

_____

_____

_____

_____

_____

What I Wish I Said

_____

_____

_____

_____

_____

_____

_____

_____

FUNNY MEMORIES

Who: _____

When: _____

To: _____

With: _____

Story/Situation

_____

_____

_____

_____

_____

What Was Said

_____

_____

_____

_____

_____

_____

_____

What I Said/My Initial Reaction

_____

_____

_____

_____

_____

_____

What I Wish I Said

_____

_____

_____

_____

_____

_____

_____

FUNNY MEMORIES

Who: _____   When: _____

To: _____   With: _____

Story/Situation

_____

_____

_____

_____

_____

What Was Said

_____

_____

_____

_____

_____

_____

_____

What I Said/My Initial Reaction

_____

_____

_____

_____

_____

_____

What I Wish I Said

_____

_____

_____

_____

_____

_____

_____

_____

_____

FUNNY MEMORIES

Who: _____ **When:** _____

To: _____ **With:** _____

Story/Situation

_____

_____

_____

_____

_____

What Was Said

_____

_____

_____

_____

_____

_____

_____

What I Said/My Initial Reaction

_____

_____

_____

_____

_____

_____

What I Wish I Said

_____

_____

_____

_____

_____

_____

_____

_____

_____

FUNNY MEMORIES

Who: _____	When: _____
To: _____	With: _____

Story/Situation

_____

_____

_____

_____

_____

What Was Said

_____

_____

_____

_____

_____

_____

_____

What I Said/My Initial Reaction

_____

_____

_____

_____

_____

_____

What I Wish I Said

_____

_____

_____

_____

_____

_____

_____

_____

_____

FUNNY MEMORIES

Who:_____   When: _____

To:_____   With: _____

Story/Situation

_____

_____

_____

_____

_____

What Was Said

_____

_____

_____

_____

_____

_____

What I Said/My Initial Reaction

_____

_____

_____

_____

_____

_____

What I Wish I Said

_____

_____

_____

_____

_____

_____

_____

_____

_____

FUNNY MEMORIES

Who: _____ | **When:** _____

To: _____ | **With:** _____

Story/Situation

_____

_____

_____

_____

_____

What Was Said

_____

_____

_____

_____

_____

_____

What I Said/My Initial Reaction

_____

_____

_____

_____

_____

_____

What I Wish I Said

_____

_____

_____

_____

_____

_____

_____

_____

FUNNY MEMORIES

Who: _____	When: _____
To: _____	With: _____

Story/Situation

_____

_____

_____

_____

_____

What Was Said

_____

_____

_____

_____

_____

_____

What I Said/My Initial Reaction

_____

_____

_____

_____

_____

_____

What I Wish I Said

_____

_____

_____

_____

_____

_____

_____

_____

FUNNY MEMORIES

Who:_____	When:_____
To:_____	With:_____

Story/Situation

_____

_____

_____

_____

_____

What Was Said

_____

_____

_____

_____

_____

_____

_____

What I Said/My Initial Reaction

_____

_____

_____

_____

_____

_____

What I Wish I Said

_____

_____

_____

_____

_____

_____

_____

_____

FUNNY MEMORIES

Who: _____	When: _____
To: _____	With: _____

Story/Situation

_____

_____

_____

_____

_____

What Was Said

_____

_____

_____

_____

_____

_____

What I Said/My Initial Reaction

_____

_____

_____

_____

_____

_____

What I Wish I Said

_____

_____

_____

_____

_____

_____

_____

_____

_____

FUNNY MEMORIES

| Who: _____ | When: _____ |
| To: _____ | With: _____ |

Story/Situation

_____

_____

_____

_____

_____

What Was Said

_____

_____

_____

_____

_____

_____

What I Said/My Initial Reaction

_____

_____

_____

_____

_____

_____

What I Wish I Said

_____

_____

_____

_____

_____

_____

_____

FUNNY MEMORIES

Who: _____	When: _____
To: _____	With: _____

Story/Situation

_____

_____

_____

_____

_____

What Was Said

_____

_____

_____

_____

_____

_____

What I Said/My Initial Reaction

_____

_____

_____

_____

_____

_____

What I Wish I Said

_____

_____

_____

_____

_____

_____

_____

_____

FUNNY MEMORIES

Who: _____   **When:** _____

To: _____   **With:** _____

Story/Situation

_____

_____

_____

_____

_____

What Was Said

_____

_____

_____

_____

_____

_____

What I Said/My Initial Reaction

_____

_____

_____

_____

_____

_____

What I Wish I Said

_____

_____

_____

_____

_____

_____

_____

_____

FUNNY MEMORIES

Who: _____   **When:** _____

To: _____   **With:** _____

Story/Situation

_____

_____

_____

_____

_____

What Was Said

_____

_____

_____

_____

_____

_____

_____

What I Said/My Initial Reaction

_____

_____

_____

_____

_____

_____

What I Wish I Said

_____

_____

_____

_____

_____

_____

_____

FUNNY MEMORIES

Who:_____	When: _____
To:_____	With: _____

Story/Situation

_____

_____

_____

_____

_____

What Was Said

_____

_____

_____

_____

_____

_____

What I Said/My Initial Reaction

_____

_____

_____

_____

_____

_____

What I Wish I Said

_____

_____

_____

_____

_____

_____

_____

_____

FUNNY MEMORIES

Who: _____	When: _____
To: _____	With: _____

Story/Situation

_____

_____

_____

_____

_____

What Was Said

_____

_____

_____

_____

_____

_____

What I Said/My Initial Reaction

_____

_____

_____

_____

_____

_____

What I Wish I Said

_____

_____

_____

_____

_____

_____

_____

_____

FUNNY MEMORIES

Who: _____	When: _____
To: _____	With: _____

Story/Situation

_____

_____

_____

_____

_____

What Was Said

_____

_____

_____

_____

_____

_____

What I Said/My Initial Reaction

_____

_____

_____

_____

_____

_____

What I Wish I Said

_____

_____

_____

_____

_____

_____

_____

_____

FUNNY MEMORIES

Who: _____

When: _____

To: _____

With: _____

Story/Situation

_____

_____

_____

_____

_____

What Was Said

_____

_____

_____

_____

_____

_____

What I Said/My Initial Reaction

_____

_____

_____

_____

_____

_____

What I Wish I Said

_____

_____

_____

_____

_____

_____

_____

_____

FUNNY MEMORIES

| Who: _____ | When: _____ |
| To: _____ | With: _____ |

Story/Situation

_____

_____

_____

_____

_____

What Was Said

_____

_____

_____

_____

_____

_____

_____

What I Said/My Initial Reaction

_____

_____

_____

_____

_____

_____

What I Wish I Said

_____

_____

_____

_____

_____

_____

_____

_____

FUNNY MEMORIES

Who: _____	**When:** _____
To: _____	**With:** _____

Story/Situation

_____

_____

_____

_____

_____

What Was Said

_____

_____

_____

_____

_____

_____

_____

What I Said/My Initial Reaction

_____

_____

_____

_____

_____

_____

What I Wish I Said

_____

_____

_____

_____

_____

_____

_____

_____

FUNNY MEMORIES

Who: _____   **When:** _____

To: _____   **With:** _____

Story/Situation

_____

_____

_____

_____

_____

What Was Said

_____

_____

_____

_____

_____

_____

What I Said/My Initial Reaction

_____

_____

_____

_____

_____

_____

What I Wish I Said

_____

_____

_____

_____

_____

_____

_____

FUNNY MEMORIES

| Who: _____ | When: _____ |
| To: _____ | With: _____ |

Story/Situation

_____

_____

_____

_____

_____

What Was Said

_____

_____

_____

_____

_____

_____

_____

What I Said/My Initial Reaction

_____

_____

_____

_____

_____

_____

What I Wish I Said

_____

_____

_____

_____

_____

_____

_____

_____

FUNNY MEMORIES

Who: _____	When: _____
To: _____	With: _____

Story/Situation

_____

_____

_____

_____

_____

What Was Said

_____

_____

_____

_____

_____

_____

What I Said/My Initial Reaction

_____

_____

_____

_____

_____

_____

What I Wish I Said

_____

_____

_____

_____

_____

_____

_____

FUNNY MEMORIES

Who: _____	When: _____
To: _____	With: _____

Story/Situation

_____

_____

_____

_____

_____

What Was Said

_____

_____

_____

_____

_____

_____

_____

What I Said/My Initial Reaction

_____

_____

_____

_____

_____

_____

What I Wish I Said

_____

_____

_____

_____

_____

_____

_____

FUNNY MEMORIES

Who: _____	When: _____
To: _____	With: _____

Story/Situation

_____

_____

_____

_____

_____

What Was Said

_____

_____

_____

_____

_____

_____

What I Said/My Initial Reaction

_____

_____

_____

_____

_____

_____

What I Wish I Said

_____

_____

_____

_____

_____

_____

_____

_____

FUNNY MEMORIES

Who:_____   **When:**_____

To:_____   **With:**_____

Story/Situation

_____

_____

_____

_____

_____

What Was Said

_____

_____

_____

_____

_____

_____

_____

What I Said/My Initial Reaction

_____

_____

_____

_____

_____

_____

What I Wish I Said

_____

_____

_____

_____

_____

_____

_____

_____

FUNNY MEMORIES

Who: _____ **When:** _____

To: _____ **With:** _____

Story/Situation

_____

_____

_____

_____

_____

What Was Said

_____

_____

_____

_____

_____

_____

_____

What I Said/My Initial Reaction

_____

_____

_____

_____

_____

_____

_____

What I Wish I Said

_____

_____

_____

_____

_____

_____

_____

_____

_____

Printed in Great Britain
by Amazon

72228832R00059